Slimability

by
JACQUELYN LOU BRADLEY

AuthorHouse™
1663 Liberty Drive, Suite 200
Bloomington, IN 47403
www.authorhouse.com
Phone: 1-800-839-8640

First published by AuthorHouse   1/21/2008

ISBN: 978-1-4343-3463-3 (sc)

Library of Congress Control Number: 2007907033

Printed in the United States of America
Bloomington, Indiana

This book is printed on acid-free paper.

I would like to first give God the Glory for giving me the ability to lose weight and enjoy life.

Slimability is designed to help you loose weight through the divine wisdom of God.

There are many man made products and stimulates on the market that can assist in weight loss and some are very successful. But if you prefer to loose weight naturally and develop a lifestyle of eating properly, then you have chosen the right book to aid you in your weight loss journey.

I would like to encourage you to love yourself and think good about yourself, no matter what weight you are today. You don't have to be a fashion model or look like you just stepped out of G-Q Magazine in order to be healthy. Enjoy who you are and make the best of you that is possible. I encourage you to loose all the weight you need and not settle for half your goal. The Scriptures says" Beloved I wish above all things that thou mayest prosper and be in good health, even as thy soul prosper. God wants you healthy and wealthy and for you to have a healthy mindset as well.

Remember that your body is your access to this world; if you don't take care of your body you will not live out all your days. In the Old Testament, men lived to be hundreds of years old; but in our society today, we have moved so far away from eating right and because we have allowed sin to reign in our mortal bodies; mankind days have been cut short. God does desire that every person live to enjoy at least 70 years of life or greater. This book will help you prolong your life span and enjoy the power of eternal life on the inside of you. You are special and God loves you. Keep these thoughts in your head as you journey down the Road to healthy eating and weight loss success.

This book can help anyone, male and female alike. Whether you want to get back into that size 8 dress, for the women or have a 32-inch waistline for the men; your desired goals can be accomplished by practicing these few simple, but powerful techniques. When you began to read this book don't forget to turn to the back of the book and utilize the chart to record your beginning weight. This is a very important step in your weight loss journey. Well, its time to get started.

May God bless you in your endeavor to loose weight, and cause you to live a long and prosperous life.

Table of Contents

Chapter I
Slimability

This book is intended to help you realize that you have the power within you to become slim or to reach your desired weight loss and to maintain it.

Let me give you a brief testimony of myself in my battle of the bulge, the fight against obesity and how I am winning, even today as I write this book.

TESTIMONY

It was in February 2003, that after 10 years of fighting the obesity war and losing it;

I decided to take this matter to the Lord in prayer. Not that I had not prayed before about this matter, but I would always try things that was out on the market and thought my efforts alone would bring success. I decided to stop trying to win this battle on my own. I tried just about every diet fad out there; from diet pills to patches, you name it, I probably tried it. I did experience limited success, but not success that were lasting. From my studies of the bible, I knew that God is the maker of all mankind and that Psalm 139 tells us that we are uniquely and wonderfully made. With this mindset, this inspired me to pray and ask for guidance in losing weight. God knows you more than anyone else and He alone is the designer of this human body with its complex make-up. Just like anything else in our society today, if it is not working properly, we take it back to the manufacturer or where is it was purchased, to get a resolution to the problem. Likewise, when we don't function right, we can go to the God who created us. So this is what I did. I was so afraid of being overweight all my life, and I found out the more I feared being fat the fatter I got.

As I sought God's help, he began to reveal to me that I had a failure spirit called fear operating in my life and that it caused major malfunction to my efforts to fighting the obesity war. For a little while I would do good, but ultimately I would go back to binge eating again. See fear was not designed for the human body, it's an evil spirit and causes men hearts to fail and not meet their destiny in life. I was also afraid of sickness and diseases coming on my body from being obese. So I realized, I needed to be healed from a failure spirit of fear. The second thing that the Lord showed me was that I had a spirit of Greed and Gluttony operating in my life. Greed is desiring more than your portion needed of any one thing and gluttony is living without boundaries or riotous living. This two spirits influenced the way I ate or thought about food. Eating more than the designated portion and eating without restrains, cause my body to experience obesity. The Lord gave me the remedy to having the spirit of failure, fear, greed and gluttony. First thing I had to do was repent for allowing these spirits operation in my life and ask God to cleanse me from these unrighteous spirits. See God is a Spirit, and he operates in the Spirit realm.

He is spirit and truth. He is the only wise God. He is the maker of Heaven and Earth. No one can rule Him or outdo Him. He is the most Supernatural force in the entire world. And most of all He loves us and wants us to win in every aspect of life. He however is not pleased when He sees an unclean spirit in our lives, for we were created in his own image and in his likeness (Genesis 1:26). So as I sought God, he required me to repent for the unclean spirits in my life. Repentance is a pronouncing or admitting fault and then turning away from the act of sin. God will only accept true worship from all of us. If you are not experiencing victory in your life, please examine your worship unto God. In the flesh realm or sin realm we cannot please God.

As I Looked at the operation of God, even in our natural surroundings, He spoke a world into existence according to Genesis 1:1. Then recreated a world in

Genesis 1:2. This world still stands today. The moon still shines at night and the sun still shines by day. With this track record, I am willing to believe what He has to say to fix any malfunction or ailment within me. His word states in 1 John 1:9, that if I confess my sins, He is faithful and just to forgive me and cleanse me from all unrighteousness. He will forgive sin and take them away. After the confession of having foreign spirits influencing me, the Lord God instructed me on a 3 day fast. For some things come only through fasting and prayer. Matthew 17:21. Upon the finish of the 3-day fast, I began to see that the spirits of fear, greed and gluttony, no longer had influence over me. My thoughts were different and much peace was upon. He measured me faith, ignited patience and temperance in me, to get the job done. All this was made possible because of the Spirit of Christ that lives within me. For he hath made him to be sin for us, who knew no sin; that we might be made the righteousness of God in him. (II Corinthians. 5:21). See Jesus was made to carry your sin and bear the punishment also, so that you and I can live a peaceful life unto God through him. I am now free from lust of the flesh, lust of the eye and the pride life. Jesus is the remedy to my obesity problem. I am now free from the influence of evil spirits and their desires in my life. I can now pay attention to restoration methods of weight loss in my life. Like proper eating and exercise.

This weight loss method works for those who have His spirit working in them. To get God's Spirit working in you, you must acknowledge Jesus as Lord and that you have sinned against God. See the prayer in the following chapter to make this wonderful transition happen in your life.

Finally, He then began to instruct me on how to eat proper portions and exercise daily. What a freedom to have, I began to loose weight immediately. After my first night at the gym and eating right portions of the right foods, I saw a 3-pound weight loss overnight. From then on the weight has continued to drop. I have lost a total of 55 pounds and plan to loose another 30.

The key to this is that when I approached God with this problem, He went right to the root of the problem and solved it. Because his spirit gives life, He gave me the ability to loose weight and change my eating habits through the knowledge I have gained.

I am know enjoying living longer and am now 6-dress size smaller than I was before I began this journey. I have about 3 dress sizes to go to meet my goal. I am winning the battle of obesity, because I'm free from binding evil influences of fear, failure, greed and gluttony; (the law of sin and death), and now I'm experiencing love, faith, peace, temperance (the law of life in Christ Jesus).

For the law of life in Christ Jesus (the life giving power), sets me free from the law of sin and death (that which causes me to die due to the sins of myself or sins of others).

You can read more about theses evil influences and the great love that God gives us by his Spirit in the book of Galatians the 5th chapter.

Having a relationship with God through Jesus Christ is the best place to be in life. It's like having the CEO of the entire world as your very own Father. You get can get what you ask for, if you are asking for the right thing.

You can trust God to fix whatever is out of order in your life. Just trust Him. Psalm 3:5

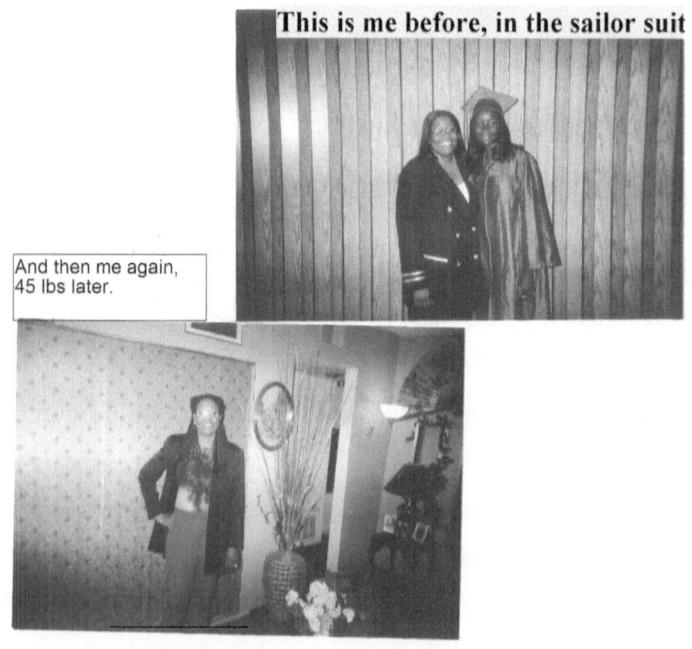

This is me before, in the sailor suit

And then me again, 45 lbs later.

Chapter II
Getting Ready

As we go along in this chapter, there are some principles that you must practice if you plan or intend to do weight lose at its finest; that is without the help of drugs or mind altering substance. In this chapter I will also share the successful things that our creator (Jehovah God), has given me that caused me to lose weight effectively. If you are sincere about your health and really want to get into shape, then you have chosen the right book.

It does not matter if you what to loose 10 pounds of 100 pounds; these techniques will work for you. I must warn you though, on this journey, your main ingredient for this success is Faith and Spiritual Warfare. We often hear that as Americans, we fight the battle of the bulge. That is a true statement, we must fight to obtain our health in this society. According to statistics, obesity has reached its highest point within the last decade. There is more obesity among our children now more than ever. There is more all-you-can -eat places today than ever. With the accessibility to these types of places, that serve food without defining the right portion, and all boundaries removed, no restraints are enforced as to how much food you can eat; it's no wonder we are a generation of fat people. Temperance or moderation is not normally exercised in these types of places and if you want to be successful in your weight loss, please avoid these places as much as possible. To me it's much like riotous living; no boundaries, no limits.

There is a constant battle to win our health in our world today. We must stand for our right to be healthy, just as we stand for our right to be free.

The way to success in these bodies is to find out how this complex system works. The way to fix anything that is broken is to take it back to the manufacturer, or the inventor of the item or product. The way to get health in these bodies and win the of obesity, is to go back to God, our creator. What better way to find out how he intended for us to live in these bodies and how they are to function. Before you put this book down thinking that this is some type of hoax or some spiritual fanatic speaking; continue to read and your reward will be great.

Lets look at our Creator God in the book of Genesis 1:26, " And God Said, Let us make man in our own image, after our likeness, and let them have dominion over the fish of the sea, and over the fowl of the air, over the cattle, and over all the earth, and over every creeping thing that creepeth upon the earth. Verse 27, so God created man in his own image, in the image of God created he him; male and female.

So, we now see that the highest form of any being made us; that is God himself.

We can trust God to lead us and direct us, because he made us. He knows exactly how our bodies are made and what it takes to maintain it in a healthy way. He even knows everything about you; for Psalms 139, tell s us that He is acquainted with all our ways. He knows our down sitting and our uprising. This means God knows what makes you tick, and he knows the thoughts that you think, and he is aware of everything that concerns you. More importantly He cares and He loves you.

In order for this process to be successful in your life, you must acknowledge Him as God, and except His way of doing things. Let's do first things first. Let acknowledge Jesus as the Son of God and repent for living a life without Him as Lord of your life. The Holy Scriptures says" I am the way, the truth and the life; no man cometh to the Father, but by me. Jesus is the way to the Father, and the Father is your way to success.

If you are already a Christian, then you merely need to repent of the spirit of fear, failure, gluttony and Greed (or anything else he reveals to you), and ask God to cleanse you and direct your path to proper eating for your life.

HERE ARE CONFESSIONS TO HELP

YOU IN YOUR PRAYER TO GOD.

FIRST TIME CONFESSORS

Dear Heavenly Father, I come to you in the name of Jesus and ask for forgiveness of living a life without you. I believe that you sent Jesus to die for my sins and bring me back in to correct relationship with you. I except Jesus as Lord of my life, (which means I except being saved from all that would come to destroy my life, including myself). Thank you for forgiving me and restoring me back to you; my Creator. Bless me with the strength and the power to overcome obesity and live the life you intended for me to live. Please return me to the health and wealth that you have planned for my life. In Jesus name. Amen.

CONFESSION FOR THE BELIEVER

Dear heavenly Father, I come in the name of Jesus, and repent for the sins of Gluttony and Greed and any iniquity and sins found in me. I John 1:9 state: If we confess our sins, He is faithful and just to forgive me and to cleanse me from all unrighteousness. I thank you for forgiveness of these and all sins in my life. Teach me the way to possess my body in holiness and to eat right. Thank you for washing me with the eternal life giving blood of Jesus Christ (that cleanses all sins) and making me strong where I was weak. I commit my ways to you and except your ways of doing things and eating properly. I will devote the time and effort to make my goal of weight loss come true. Thank you Father for making me in your image and likeness and I will and do succeed in your strength. In Jesus name. Amen

If you made either of these confessions, you are now ready to start your journey to being slim. Don't be afraid and don't doubt, because God is more willing to help you and see you succeed. His word says, " Fear not little flock (his children), it is your Father's good pleasure to give you the kingdom. God wants you to be healthy and to lose the weight that you desire. Tell God how much you desire to loose and follow his directions to get there. When you walk in the Spirit of God, He will tell you how much weight we need to lose. He knows everything about you and He knows what it will take you to look your very best.

Trust Him. Psalms 139 says that I am uniquely and wonderfully made, and that all my parts are written in his books. He knows you and what it will take to get you to your healthiest state. He may tell you directly or he may use your doctor or some other source, but he will let you know how much to loose. He will stay with you until the goal is accomplished and even after that. Being confident of this very thing, that he which hath began a good work in you will perform it until the day of Jesus Christ: (Philippians 1:6).

Trust Him

Chapter III
Knowledge is Power

Now that we are ready to get started; the next tool to add to our success is knowledge.

Applied knowledge is power. Unapplied knowledge is inactive power.

In order to be successful in anything, you must follow instructions or submit and commit to the plan to achieve your goals. You can't go off helter-skelter and expect to meet your goals. Let's gain some knowledge and apply it to our lives and win.

Knowledge comes from God and he is able to direct your path for what you need.

I Samuel 2:3 says" Talk no more exceedingly proudly; let not arrogancy come out of thy mouth; for the Lord God is a God of Knowledge, and by him actions are weighed. In other word, don't let your way of thinking and talking be above that what God has spoken for you. Humbleness is the way to the top.

King Solomon asked God for wisdom and knowledge; and God granted him that and more. (2 Chronicles1: 10). Psalms 139 states that all of our parts (our total make up) is written in his book, God knows who you are and want you need. Trust Him.

We perish for lack of knowledge. We miss out or fail for lack of knowledge.

Read materials and books that promote weight loss. Maybe subscribe or purchase magazines that promote healthy eating and good nutrition. It is very important that we learn good eating habits and are able to discern good foods from bad foods.

By his knowledge shall my righteous servant justify many. (Isaiah 52:11b)

Learn the proper eating portion for your body and incorporate proper exercise in your daily routine. Every individual is different and will vary in eating methods. Your weight loss will come easier if you now how to manage your food in take and count your calories. Calorie intake plays a great part of your weight loss and management. A balance of proper food intake and proper exercise will be needed to accomplish your weight lose.

By a calorie counting books and chart your daily food caloric intake. Join a health club, if your finances permit it or purchase exercise tapes or DVDs to work out at home.

Knowledge is power when it is applied. Attached see the Food and Exercise Log, for the daily keep of your success. You are on the right course for successful weigh loss. Experience the peace on God and the Assurance of God on your journey as you submit to Him.

WEEK ONE

Begining: _____   Starting Weight_____

	Breakfast	Morning Snack	Lunch
Monday	1 c. cantaloupe (57) 2 slices pineapple (60) instant oatmeal (100) 1 c. skim milk (90) [307]	4 rice crackers (40) 2 tsp. peanut butter (70) [110]	Low carb wrap (140) 3 oz. turkey breast (90) lettuce & tomato (40) dressing (80) [350]
Tuesday	1 c. cantaloupe (57) instant oatmeal (100) 1 c. skim milk (90) [247]	fat free yogurt (120)	Low carb wrap (140) 2 oz. light cheese (180) lettuce & tomato (40) dressing (80) [400]
Wednesday	2 slices pineapple (60) 1 c. shredded wheat (180) 1 c. skim milk (90) [330]	4 rice crackers (40) 2 tsp. peanut butter (70) [110]	Low carb wrap (140) 2 fat free franks (100) lettuce & tomato (40) [280]
Thursday	1 slice 9-grain bread (110) 1 egg (70) 1 c. skim milk (90) [180]	4 rice crackers (40) 2 tsp. peanut butter (70) [110]	Low carb wrap (140) 2 oz.light cheese (140) lettuce & tomato (40) dressing (80) [400]
Friday	1 c. mixed fruit (100) 3 slices turkey bacon (90) 1 c. skim milk (90) [280]	4 rice crackers (40) 2 tsp. peanut butter (70) [110]	Low carb wrap (140) 2 scrambled eggs (180) green pepper (18) tbsp. light butter (35) [375]
Saturday	1 c. mixed fruit (100) instant oatmeal (100) 1 c. skim milk (90) [307]	4 rice crackers (40) 2 tsp. peanut butter (70) [110]	Low carb wrap (140) 3 oz. turkey breast (90) lettuce & tomato (40) dressing (80) [350]
Sunday	1 peach (40) 1 c. shredded wheat (170) 1 c. skim milk (90) [307]	fat free yogurt (120)	2 c. salad (50) 3 oz. tuna (105) dressing (80) slice 9-grain bread (110) [345]

Afternoon Snack	Dinner	Daily Total Calories	Exercise
4 rice crackers (40) 1 oz. light cheese (70) [110]	2 fat free franks (100) slice 9-grain bread (110) c. broccoli (50) nectarine (70) [430]	1307	DVD Workout 30 min. a.m. 30 min. pool
hard-boiled egg (90)	3 oz. flounder (100) 1 c. brown rice (150) 1 c. spinach (60) 2 c. cubed watermelon (100) [410]	1267	DVD Workout 30 min. a.m. 30 min. pool
1 oz. nuts (190)	3 oz. turkey breast (90) slize 9-grain bread (110) 1 c. green beans (40) 1 c. cantaloupe (57) [297]	1207	DVD Workout 30 min. a.m. 30 min. pool
fat-free yogurt (120)	3 oz. flounder (100) 1 c. brown rice (150) 1 c. spinach (60) 2 c. cubed watermelon (100) [410]	1220	30 min. mall walk
smart pop mini bag popcorn (120)	2 fat free franks (100) slice 9-grain bread (110) c. broccoli (50) nectarine (70) [430]	1315	30 min. mall walk 30 min. pool
4 rice crackers (40) 1 oz. light cheese (70) [110]	2 c. salad (50) 3 oz. tuna (105) dressing (80) slice 9-grain bread (110) [345]	1222	DVD Workout 30 min. a.m. 30 min. pool
smart pop mini bag popcorn (120)	2 fat free franks (100) slice 9-grain bread (110) c. broccoli (50) nectarine (70) [430]	1322	DVD Workout 30 min. a.m. 30 min. pool

Jacquelyn Lou Bradley

You are uniquely and Wonderfully made, you can do all things through Christ which has strengthen you. Let the weak say I am strong; let the poor say I am rich.

Example of Calorie intake is 1200-1500 calorie a day. Any weight loss website can instruct you on the amount of calories a day you should intake. If you cannot locate one, please email me at <u>Bradley Jacqueline @yahoo.com</u>, and I will be glad to assist you in finding the proper caloric intake needed for you through qualified resources.

8/15/2005

To loose 35 pounds I need to eat 1200 calories a day and exercise and burn at least 300 calories a day.

Diet Plan		calorie count
Breakfast		
soup		175
1/2 apple or 4 cubed 2 inch or watermelon		40
1/2 orange		40
8 oz. skim milk		90
16 oz of water		0
	total	345
Snack	10:30pm	
1/2 apple		40
1 cup cucumbers		40
8 oz of water		0
	total	80
Lunch		
2 cups salad		60
5 oz tuna		150
1/2 soup		100
1/2 apple		40
	total	350
Snack	3:30pm	
1/2 orange		40
1 cup cucumbers		40
8oz water		0
	total	80
Dinner		
1 can green beans		90
4 oz of fish or turkey ot chicken		180
16 oz water		
	total	270
	Daily Calorie Consumption	1125

Exercise program burning 200-300 calories a day.

90 day program

Chart your weight daily   162

Chapter IV
Building your Faith

Now its time to determine how much weight we want to loose and be specific with the numbers. We can ask The Father our manufacturer, how much weight we need to loose to be healthy. We are not trying to look like a fashion model or be a size 2 overnight, but we want a plan that workable and sensible to give us a healthy body to live in and to enjoy life in. Your body is your passage way into earth, and if you don't take care of it, you will not enjoy the life God mean for you to have nor enjoy the length of days god has for you to live (minimum 70 years).

First we need to determine what is a healthy body weight for you and a sensible goal for you to meet. Don't try to go to fast, but let the fruit of longsuffering coupled with your faith, help you reach your goal. Do your research and find out how much weight you should be for your body build and for your height. Any health publication or health oriented internet web page can help you determine your correct body size. I utilized www.caloriecountercharts.com, to obtain information of how much I should weigh and how many calories I should intake only daily basis to remain healthy. It even shows you how many calories to reduce in your food intake to reach your appointed goal. Obtaining knowledge before hand will help you better reach your goal, for without a plan you will fail. For instance, if your body weight is 200 and you are five feet 10 inches tall, you probably would be at your best weight at 155 pounds. That means you need to loose at least 45 pounds to be at your right body weight.

So, with the information you should start changing your eating habits to produce 45 pounds of weight loss. Secondly, we must find the right foods that will help us reach our goal. For instance, fiber is needed to burn fat and produce weight loss. Fruits and vegetables are a great source of fiber. Fiber causes the body to breakdown fat cells, resulting in weight loss. Lean meats also are a good source of nutrition and will help also in weight loss. Too many fatty foods and sugary foods will not work on your weight loss plan. These are foods for pleasure to the soul and will deceive you and defeat your purpose of weight loss. You must know that only when you walk in truth shall you be free. Don't lie to your self or defend your own greed, but do what is best for your body to cause better health and a long life. Read health books, and/or magazines, listen to health talk shows and healthy cooking shows to gain tips on what foods would work best with your weight loss plan.

Here is the Soup Plan that I used to produce weight loss in my life.

Jackie's Champion Soups

2 cans of Diced tomatoes (not stewed)

2 cans of green beans

2 cans of diced carrots

½ stalk of green onions

1 package of Lipton Onion soup mix

1 can of beef broth (chicken or vegetable)

Water to cover all vegetables

Broccoli

Collie Flower

Garlic powder

Celery (if desired)

Put all contents in a large pot and stir until mixed well.

Let this cook approx. 30 minutes are until vegetables are well steamed.

Let cool and serve.

If you must have protein, you can add lima beans, dark red kidney beans, shrimp, scallops or small fish pieces. This soup can be prepared in varies ways. I would recommend eating at one bowl with every meal for at least the first 2 months of working your faith. This soup base serves as a **destroyer** of your fat cells and a **booster** to your metabolism. As well as an anti-dioxide for your inner organs.

BUILDING YOUR FAITH

Food Preparation is another area we have to change to create weight loss.

If you are accustomed to lots of seasonings or meat seasonings you will have to cut back on these items. Most seasonings have salt, which causes water retention, which results in weight gain. And most meats used for seasonings carry too much salt. Like smoked ham, or ham hocks. Try using smoke turkey in moderation to lessen your salt intake. It may help if you are going to eat this type of foods to eat it at lunch time, that way you have more time for the body to burn the excess salt intake. And Please follow this meal with a tall glass of water, to flush your system. I would recommend, lean meats like: turkey, tuna, and chicken (no fried foods). Hold off on the red meats until you have reached at least have your goal. Red meats contain many fat grams, usually more so than other meats, and have a tendency to stay in your system a lot longer than other meats.

Watch your **flour intake**. This will increase the fat cell size. Normally causing fat cells to swell or bloat, if not eaten in moderation. The name of the game is to decrease the fat cell size and not to increase it. **Fat begets fat**.

Flour breaks down into sugar in your body and if you don't exercise and burn this substance, it turns into **fat.** Starchy foods such as potatoes, rice, and pasta can cause the same increase of fat cells, if not eaten in moderation. Eat small portions of these foods.

Sugar is probably your number one enemy in fighting the weight loss battle.

Sugar is not good for the body, because the body can't naturally break it down, so it must be burned through the form of exercise. Did you know that approximately 10 grams of sugar could hinder your immune system from functioning at it fullest capacity? And it also works against your metabolism. Try using honey instead of sugar, it's a natural and the body can process honey.

Well, you are probably saying, " well what can I eat to enjoy myself"?

My answer is that you are not eating for enjoyment first, you are eating to correct your bad habits and to gain control of your appetite, which in turn will result in your weight loss, not only for know, but you will have these good eating habits built-in your way of life, for the rest of your life.

Your enjoyment will come, when you gain the confidence to become

Healthy and enjoy the life that you were intended to have.

Your priorities will be in place and then you choose what foods you will enjoy that will not alter your weight loss and health success. You are winning then game and enjoying food, when **<u>you are controlling your desires for food and not food controlling you and your desires.</u> Last but not least, don't forget your vitamins.**

Consult your doctor as to what type of vitamins are sufficient for you.

Caloric Intake Log

Breakfast_____

Caloric intake_____

Mid Morning Snack_____

Caloric Intake_____

Lunch_____

Caloric Intake_____

Mid Afternoon Snack_____

Caloric Intake_____

Supper_____

Caloric Intake_____

Total calories for today_____

Exercise_____

How many calories burned?_____

You did great, now lets do it again.

Record your activities daily, keep sharp and keep alert.
You are more than a conqueror, you are a winner!

WEEKLY FOOD CHART

Begining: _____   Starting Weight_____

	Breakfast	Morning Snack	Lunch
Monday			
Tuesday			
Wednesday			
Thursday			
Friday			
Saturday			
Sunday			

Afternoon Snack	Dinner	Daily Total Calories	Exercise

Chapter V
Working Your Faith

Faith without its works is dead. We can't merely wish for weight loss, we must apply the knowledge we have learned in to action. Then we become what we hope for. Faith is the substance of things hoped for and the evidence of things not seen. We have visualized the amount of weigh we want to loose, but now we must walk out our vision to make it sight.

Let's take our measurements first and record them. Having record of you starting point will cause you to be encouraged as you see you inch reductions come about as you began to work your faith.

Measurement Chart

Today's date of measurements_____

Measurements

:

Right Arm_____Left Arm_____

Chest Area_____ Waist Line_____
Hips_____

Right Thigh_____Left Thigh_____

At the end of every two to three weeks measure yourself and chart your results from eating and exercising. (Working your faith).

Measurement Chart

About 2 or 3 Weeks after your first measurements take them again and chart your success. And again and again until you get to the size you desire. This can be done once a month or once a week, whatever is best for you to stay encouraged.

Today's date of measurements_____

Measurements

:

Right Arm_____Left Arm_____

Chest Area_____ Waist Line_____

Hips_____

Right Thigh_____Left Thigh_____

You are doing great! Keep it up!

Today's date of measurements_____

Measurements

:

Right Arm_____Left Arm_____

Chest Area_____ Waist Line_____
Hips_____
Right Thigh_____Left Thigh_____

LOOK AT THE RESULTS OF YOUR
FAITH WOW! KEEP MOVING

Today's date of measurements_____

Measurements

:

Right Arm_____Left Arm_____

Chest Area_____ Waist Line_____
Hips_____
Right Thigh_____Left Thigh_____

YOUR GREATNESS IS SHINNING THROUGH! YOU LOOK GREAT!
Make copies of this page as often as you need too.

WORKING YOUR FAITH

Let's look at another area that is essential to your weight loss success.

That is your consumption of drinking water.

The body is made up of 95% water. Water keeps your organs, skin, hair, muscle, and eyes healthy. It works on every part of your body. Insufficient water intake can affect your thinking ability also. Dehydration is a negative return on your investment for good health.

Drinking juices verses water is not good for you when you are seeking to loose weight.

Some fruit juices contain too much sugar and will affect your ability to loose the weight, as you should. Carbonated drinks also detour your weight loss. If you desire a soft drink or soda, please drink a sugar free drink. Sodas are not good for your overall health either, for they eventually deteriorate the bones. Especially for women over 35 years of age, you should be careful of your soda intake, so that you can promote healthy bone structure through your menopause stage; which is known to decrease your bone density in some women. So try to stay with Purified Drinking Water in the bottle. Buying bottled water vs. drinking tap water is better for your health. Bottled water is cleaner and don't have any additives that may harm your health in general. Whereas, tap water has not gone though the purifying stages and may have an affect on the body after drinking it over a period of time. Not always, but it is best to have bottled water to maintain good health.

So DRINK UP. WATER, WATER,

AND MORE WATER!

You should try to consume at least 64 ounces of water daily. That's 8 eight-ounce glasses.

If you are not accustomed to drinking water, you may say that is a lot of water to drink, but let me show you how to do it.

First, when you get up in the morning drink an 8-ounce glass of water, then with your breakfast drink another 8 ounces. With you mid morning snack drink another 8 ounces; with lunch drink 8 more ounces, with your afternoon snack drink 16 ounces of water, with dinner drink 16 ounces of water and 8 ounces with your evening snack. That is equivalent to 64 ounces a day. Now that does not seem to hard after you break it down does it?

Working Your Faith

Now that you have decided how much weight you want to loose, now we must apply the work to go with your faith. Faith without works is dead. We can't make a statement and then not put some action behind it to make the statement a reality. We must WORK our faith. WORK - Winning On Real Knowledge.

You have obtained the information or knowledge you need to win the battle of obesity.

NOW WE MUST WALK IT OUT.

Step 1. Process your faith by exercising.

Walking is a great form of exercise. It is low impact to the knees, but excellent for the heart and the rest of the body. Daily walking will also correct your body's metabolism; which enable the body to burn fat. On e of the most important keys to weight lose, is to get the body to burn fat, and increasing your metabolism rate is the way to go. Walking also brings oxygen to the body that helps stimulate your metabolism also. A treadmill is an excellent way to walk if you can't get outside to a walking trial in a park or in your neighborhood. You **must** invest time into your health. Take about 30-45 minutes daily it invest into better health. If you know anything about investments you know there is a return on your principle if invested in the right way. Well, you can count on a return from your time invested in your health. For example if you invest 45 minutes of walking with a little brisk to it, you can burn approximately 300-350 calories. If this is done at least 4 to 5 days of the week, you will receive a return of weight lost and a reduction if inches through out your body. GREAT RETURNS on your investment. The more you invest your time in to exercise, the bigger your returns will be. So let's get started so that we can finish our course.

Working your faith

Another form of exercise is the bicycle. Whether it is mobile or a stationary bike.

Investing about 30 minutes on a bicycle daily will give you great returns on your stomach, hips, buttocks and thighs.

You can burn several hundreds of calories from bike riding. If you bike alone a trail, please try to take a friend with you if possible. With the crime rate in our society today we must be careful of our surroundings. Practice safety while you are on your weight loss success journey. You should see considerable inch reduction from you bicycling activities. If you go to a local gym to work out this could work to your advantage. ON some machines, you can program the machine for the amount time you choose to invest in your health and it will tell you how many calories per hour you can expect to burn from cycling. This is a way to keep up with your fat burning number to record in your daily log to chart your progress. Remember to count your caloric in take and to count you fat burned calories also. This is a very important component to your weight loose success. If you over eat and do little exercise you will receive a negative return on your investment which will cause disappointment. So remember to eat right, stay within your calorie intake and keep your fat burning up daily to receive a position return on your investments.

WORKING YOUR FAITH

Another form of exercise is **Aerobics.** Low or high impact, whatever is best for you. Don't to forget t consult with your physician before exercising if you have any medical problems. Get advice on the best exercise for your condition. Aerobics can burn several hundreds of calories also, and tone your body at the same time. You can purchase any low or impact aerobic exercise video from any local bookstore or grocer. I have seen a variety of exercise programs on CDs at Wal-Mart or Target. Be sure you get what is best for your health. Your age and beginning weight should be a determining factor as to what type of aerobic exercise you should partake in.

Remember that you are making an Investment into your health and future. Get good returns on your time invested into aerobics exercising.

Inspiration: Take out an old dress or pants that you used to wear, that maybe to small for you now, or purchase a dress or pants that maybe two or three size smaller than what you are now; and use this item as your target for return on your investment from your aerobics. Remember to give yourself time and diligence to your plan to see results.

Defeating Negative Results

There are times when you may fall off the wagon or get tempted to over eat and return to your old habits. This chapter will help you to get back on track again. Prayerfully this chapter will suit you up again with the armor to fight the battle of obesity.

What has happened, you have let down your guard or shield of protection, or you have had a change in mindset to alter your weight loss success. This could come from a loss of a job or income, a temptation succumbed to, a break up of a relationship, the enduring a bad relationship, or a loss of a loved one etc... There could be many reason for disappointments in our lives, but we must remember that you are in control of your health and no one else, besides God Himself. You are supposed to have good health. 3 John in the bible tells us "beloved I wish above all things that you may prosper and be in health, even as your soul prospers. Good health belongs to you. Defend your God given right to be healthy and stay healthy.

Forgive your self for the mistakes you make and get up and try again. Don't let negative results of not exercising or eating outside of your designed food group, stop you from trying again. The only way to complete failure is to stop trying. As long as you keep trying you will meet success.

Let me encourage you in your faith. Your faith is so powerful that it can create a whole New World for you. If we go back to the beginning, where faith comes from; and see the effect that faith had on the world we live in, we can better hold on to our faith and make our destiny. Let's look at how God used faith at the making of this world. Genesis 1:1-2 states that in the beginning God created the heaven and the earth. And the earth was without form and void, and darkness was upon the face of the deep. And God the Spirit of God moved upon the face of the waters. And God said Let there be light", and there was light, And God saw the light that it was good: God spoke in faith to a world that was out of order and dark and bought light to the situation and then began to speak by faith the rest of the creation. Think about this, the same light that God called or spoke has been in manifestation since the beginning of time. It always does its job and it never fails. Sure there are days that the sun does not shine, that is when we see rain clouds. That is so the earth can be cleansed and refreshed to keep producing and/or to produce more fruit. There will be days that you won't feel like exercising or days that come to make things dark in your life, please remember to continue to speak your faith that has been given to you by God and defend your success, and get back on track. Keep speaking your weight loss goal, and change or modify your eating habits to reflect your faith spoken. You being made in his image and in his likeness can also speak to your dark situation of obesity and bring light into your detoured situation. Your have not lost the battle, you are just delayed a little. Keep on your shield of faith and protect your success. This is the victory that you have even your faith. PROTECT, SPEAK, and MANIFEST.

KEEP ON YOUR SHIELD OF FAITH, FIGHT

AND KEEP WINNING THE VICTORY.

VICTORY BELONGS TO YOU!

CALORIC INTAKE LOG

Breakfast_____

Caloric intake_____

Mid Morning Snack_____

Caloric Intake_____

Lunch_____

Caloric Intake_____

Mid Afternoon Snack_____

Caloric Intake_____

Supper_____

Caloric Intake_____

Total calories for today_____

Exercise_____

How many calories burned?_____

YOU DID GREAT, NOW LETS DO IT AGAIN.

RECORD YOUR ACTIVITIES DAILY, KEEP SHARP AND KEEP ALERT.

YOU ARE MORE THAN A CONQUEROR, YOU ARE A WINNER!

Jacquelyn Lou Bradley

CALORIC INTAKE LOG

Breakfast_____

Caloric intake_____

Mid Morning Snack_____

Caloric Intake_____

Lunch_____

Caloric Intake_____

Mid Afternoon Snack_____

Caloric Intake_____

Supper_____

Caloric Intake_____

Total calories for today_____

Exercise_____

How many calories burned?_____

YOU DID GREAT, NOW LETS DO IT AGAIN.
RECORD YOUR ACTIVITIES DAILY, KEEP SHARP AND KEEP ALERT.
YOU ARE MORE THAN A CONQUEROR, YOU ARE A WINNER!

Chapter VI
Celebrate you and New life

Our next step in weight loss success is to acknowledge God for all that he has done for you. You have all the ingredients to make successful weight loss happen in your life.

We have first acknowledged God as our source of strength and life, and then we added knowledge to our faith; now we add celebrating your new life and success with praising him into our mixture to complete and sustain the outcome of victory. Celebrate your newness of life, dance, have fun, take a night of enjoyment at movie and/or dinner (but watch what you eat). Rejoice in your newfound success.

Praising God is very essential to your success also. How to praise God. We can praise him in a dance, with a shout of joy, with a handclap, showing love to others, or just telling God thank you for your new life and weight loss. Hallelujah, is the highest form of praise unto God.

Praise is a form of adoration. When we praise God, we are showing him that we adore him and that we are thankful to him for giving us power to get health.

Psalms 100 tells us to make a joyful noise unto the Lord all ye lands. Serve the Lord gladness; come before his presence with thanksgiving and enter his courts with praise.

Know ye that the Lord he is God: it is he that has made us and not we ourselves; we are the sheep of his pasture. Give God praises or adoration for what he has done and for what he will do in your life.

Praise releases you from all fear of your opponents and obstacles in your life.

Praising God also brings His presence and power into your life to handle whatever the situation or circumstances you is facing. With his power and presence, we can do miraculous things and breakdown barriers that keep us from going to the next level in life. God is omnipotent and omniscience; keeping the Father God as your focus and your supplier to your success will give you the support and help you need to accomplish your goal. Praising God will undo the mind of failure and help you to overcome temptations to overeat. Praising God will undo the work of the devil.

Keep moving in your weight loss venture, even when you miss it or binge out. Get up from your mistakes and keep moving. God has forgiven you of your sins and everything that will cause you failure. We are human and we will make mistakes. If you find the urge to eat ice cream and you happen to succumb to eat; eat a small portion and put the rest away. Don't beat yourself up if you fall, get up and praise God and he will give you more strength for the next time and for the journey.

Daily Affirmation

We must confess our goals to ourselves daily. It is good to say them out loud. This will build up your faith level. For faith comes by hearing and hearing by the word of God.

For instance, if your desired goal is to wear a certain dress size or pants size, then you should confess it to yourself daily. Write your vision on paper and post it in several places in your home. The more you see your vision and understand it the more you will strive to accomplish it. Here is an example of a daily affirmation.

I have slim ability on the inside of me to lose 45 pounds and keep it off. I have long life because I trust in God to give me daily; the mind and strength to over come every trap of over eating and indulging in unnecessary eating. I eat that which sufficient for the day and I exercise my body to burn calories to promote weight loss. I will wear a size 9 dress and pants or less. I will look my very best at all times. I will enjoy long life because I value my body and appreciate the body and life that God has given me. I am winning and not losing. I am reaching my goal daily and loving myself also. I strengthen my mind, soul and body, by praising God and reading his word, I keep knowledge of my endeavors, I keep track of my success. I am a winner and not loser. I will not quit; I will reach my goal. I praise God for daily success and continuous victory. In Jesus Name. Amen

Chapter VII
Walking in the Spirit

How we live are everyday life will also determine our steadfastness and ability to reach our goal. Since this weight loss method stems from God, God is love and we must live with him in love and with others in love. We must walk in the fruit of love, which manifest itself in joy, peace, longsuffering, gentleness, goodness, faith, meekness, temperance: against these manifestations are no binding of condemning power. You are free to serve God and lose weight and love others also. Sometimes in making changes we get irritable, but the peace of God and the love of God sustains our heart and mind through all of our transitioning to become better and reach our goals in life. The fruit of the Spirit will keep you in faith and longsuffering with yourself, while allowing you to be kind and patience with others also. Keep yourself in the love of God and the wicked one will not touch you. Stay away from negative talk, negative thoughts and evil thinking. Stay out of sin, for sin will hinder and stop your weight loss process from God. Sin brings separation from God. IJohn 5:18 We know that whosoever is born of God sinneth not; but he that is begotten of God keepeth himself, and that wicked one toucheth him not.

Some sins are outlined in Galatians 5:19-21. Practice living a holy life and you will always have success with this plan. Walk in the Spirit (love, freedom, joy, faith, peace, forgiveness etc…), and you will not fulfill the lust of the flesh (the old evil desires that come to ruin you like unforgiveness, hatred, stubbornness, malice, lust, anger, self pity, pride, etc…). In order to win you must stay in the love of God. Walk in the fruit if the spirit.

Chapter VIII
Watch out For Pitfalls

Keep on track with your designed eating habits. Watch out for junk foods.

Use food substitutes such as: eat fruits instead of candy, eat more vegetables. Eat soups and lean meats daily. Turn off the television and walk around the block. Watch out for the all you can eat places. Remember to eat proper portions. Stay away from fatty foods, high calorie foods.

Learn to say no to those who are trying to sabotage your plans, the holidays can be survived with proper planning.

Keep your daily log of food intake.

Exercise daily.

Pray daily

Stay in the love of God.

Praise God daily.

Take vitamins daily

Drink plenty water daily, at least 64 or more oz of water.

Stop drinking sodas, eating chips, cookies and ice cream;

You have already experienced the taste of these things, they can wait for you to achieve your goals. Stay in control, remember you are the head and not the tail. You are more than a conqueror.

Keep these thoughts in mind: The Spirit of God is eternal and will always be alive and ruling, the spirit of the evil one is temporary, is already defeated, and will ultimately be destroyed.

Watch for your old habits, watch your attitude, and watch your tongue.

This has much effect on your success.

TRAPS SET FOR YOUR FAITH.

There are traps set in place to lure you away from your success.

WATCH OUT!

Here are some areas of food traps to be aware of :

SUGAR:

Sugar slows down your metabolism which affects your weight loss and it also hardens your arteries, producing bad health; like heart problems and possibly diabetes. Too much sugar is bad for your teeth and can affect your skin tone. Sugary foods are usually high in calories also. Did you know that a small strawberry milkshake can contain 400 calories of more? That's a whole meal calorie content in one drink. And that does not include the hamburger and French-fries. So by the time you eat a fast food meal, you could easily consume 1200 calories at one meal setting. FAT, FAT, FAT.

Sugar is an empty calorie and really adds no nutritional value.

Try eating fruits and vegetables instead. They are low in calorie intake, provides excellent nutrition to the body, and are enjoyable to the taste palate.

Escape the food traps!

Fried Foods & Junk Foods

Chapter IX
A Lifetime Of Slimness

Now that you have the essential tools to lose your weight and reach your targeted goal; its time to maintain the work that you have accomplished by God's power. There is a famous writer that said " To be highly effective in success; you must repeat what you have already done to get success, so that you maintain your level of success". Go back over your book again; recommit to your daily affirmation, count your caloric intake, write down your daily food intake. Keep reading materials that promote weight loss and good nutrition. Please consult your physician about any weight loss program you decide to take on. Practice your exercise routine daily. Weigh yourself weekly; make sure your clothing is not getting tighter. Watch out for the " I have arrived mentality".

Yes, You have accomplished your weight loss goal, but the work is not finished yet.

Maintain your appearance at all times and enjoy your new body size.

God will never stop empowering you to be the best you can be. He made a covenant through Jesus to never leave you nor forsake you. He promised to show us mercy.

Keep binding the spirit of gluttony and greed and loosing the Spirit of Love, temperance, faith and patience.

My prayers are with every reader of this book, that God will show his mighty power and heal you in every area of your life.

May God bless you and strengthen you daily in your success journey to weight loss.

This is a self-help book, designed to guide you in successful and everlasting weight loss.

Please write to me of your success and concerns at Bradley Jacqueline@yahoo.com.

Jacquelyn Lou Bradley

Your Caloric and Food intake Log

Remember you were created a winner!

Caloric Intake Log

Breakfast_____
Caloric intake_____

Mid Morning Snack_____
Caloric Intake_____

Lunch_____
Caloric Intake_____

Mid Afternoon Snack_____
Caloric Intake_____

Supper_____
Caloric Intake_____

Total calories for today_____

Exercise_____

How many calories burned?_____

Caloric Intake Log

Breakfast_____

Caloric intake_____

Mid Morning Snack_____

Caloric Intake_____

Lunch_____

Caloric Intake_____

Mid Afternoon Snack_____

Caloric Intake_____

Supper_____

Caloric Intake_____

Total calories for today_____

Exercise_____

How many calories burned?_____

You did great, now lets do it again.

Record your activities daily, keep sharp and keep alert.

You are more than a conqueror, you are a winner!

CALORIC INTAKE LOG

Breakfast_____

Caloric intake_____

Mid Morning Snack_____

Caloric Intake_____

Lunch_____

Caloric Intake_____

Mid Afternoon Snack_____

Caloric Intake_____

Supper_____

Caloric Intake_____

Total calories for today_____

Exercise_____

How many calories burned?_____

YOU DID GREAT, NOW LETS DO IT AGAIN.

RECORD YOUR ACTIVITIES DAILY, KEEP SHARP AND KEEP ALERT.

YOU ARE MORE THAN A CONQUEROR, YOU ARE A WINNER!

CALORIC INTAKE LOG

Breakfast_____

Caloric intake_____

Mid Morning Snack_____

Caloric Intake_____

Lunch_____

Caloric Intake_____

Mid Afternoon Snack_____

Caloric Intake_____

Supper_____

Caloric Intake_____

Total calories for today_____

Exercise_____

How many calories burned?_____

YOU DID GREAT, NOW LETS DO IT AGAIN.

RECORD YOUR ACTIVITIES DAILY, KEEP SHARP AND KEEP ALERT.

YOU ARE MORE THAN A CONQUEROR, YOU ARE A WINNER!

CALORIC INTAKE LOG

Breakfast_____

Caloric intake_____

Mid Morning Snack_____

Caloric Intake_____

Lunch_____

Caloric Intake_____

Mid Afternoon Snack_____

Caloric Intake_____

Supper_____

Caloric Intake_____

Total calories for today_____

Exercise_____

How many calories burned?_____

YOU DID GREAT, NOW LETS DO IT AGAIN.

RECORD YOUR ACTIVITIES DAILY, KEEP SHARP AND KEEP ALERT.

YOU ARE MORE THAN A CONQUEROR, YOU ARE A WINNER!

CALORIC INTAKE LOG

Breakfast_____

Caloric intake_____

Mid Morning Snack_____

Caloric Intake_____

Lunch_____

Caloric Intake_____

Mid Afternoon Snack_____

Caloric Intake_____

Supper_____

Caloric Intake_____

Total calories for today_____

Exercise_____

How many calories burned?_____

YOU DID GREAT, NOW LETS DO IT AGAIN.

RECORD YOUR ACTIVITIES DAILY, KEEP SHARP AND KEEP ALERT.

YOU ARE MORE THAN A CONQUEROR, YOU ARE A WINNER!

Jacquelyn Lou Bradley

Caloric Intake Log

Breakfast_____
Caloric intake_____

Mid Morning Snack_____
Caloric Intake_____

Lunch_____
Caloric Intake_____

Mid Afternoon Snack_____
Caloric Intake_____

Supper_____
Caloric Intake_____

Total calories for today_____

Exercise_____

How many calories burned?_____

You did great, now lets do it again.
Record your activities daily, keep sharp and keep alert.
You are more than a conqueror, you are a winner!

Caloric Intake Log

Breakfast_____

Caloric intake_____

Mid Morning Snack_____

Caloric Intake_____

Lunch_____

Caloric Intake_____

Mid Afternoon Snack_____

Caloric Intake_____

Supper_____

Caloric Intake_____

Total calories for today_____

Exercise_____

How many calories burned?_____

You did great, now lets do it again.

Record your activities daily, keep sharp and keep alert.

You are more than a conqueror, you are a winner!

CALORIC INTAKE LOG

Breakfast_____

Caloric intake_____

Mid Morning Snack_____

Caloric Intake_____

Lunch_____

Caloric Intake_____

Mid Afternoon Snack_____

Caloric Intake_____

Supper_____

Caloric Intake_____

Total calories for today_____

Exercise_____

How many calories burned?_____

YOU DID GREAT, NOW LETS DO IT AGAIN.

RECORD YOUR ACTIVITIES DAILY, KEEP SHARP AND KEEP ALERT.

YOU ARE MORE THAN A CONQUEROR, YOU ARE A WINNER!

Caloric Intake Log

Breakfast_____

Caloric intake_____

Mid Morning Snack_____

Caloric Intake_____

Lunch_____

Caloric Intake_____

Mid Afternoon Snack_____

Caloric Intake_____

Supper_____

Caloric Intake_____

Total calories for today_____

Exercise_____

How many calories burned?_____

You did great, now lets do it again.

Record your activities daily, keep sharp and keep alert.

You are more than a conqueror, you are a winner!

References

References: The Holy Bible

Covey, Steve, Seven habits of highly effective people,

Web Site, www.caloriecountercharts.com

Web Site, www.caloriecontrol.org

www.ingramcontent.com/pod-product-compliance
Lightning Source LLC
Chambersburg PA
CBHW021238280526
45784CB00005B/2148